I0711449

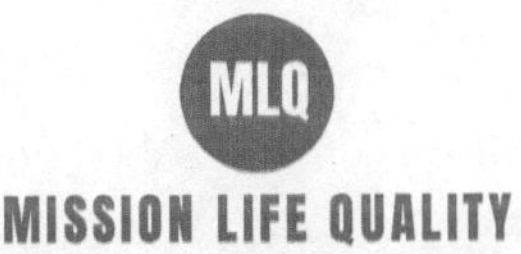

MLQ
MISSION LIFE QUALITY

HABITS
FOR
SUCCESS

ALL YOU NEED TO KNOW ABOUT HABITS TO TAKE FULL CONTROL OF YOUR LIFE AND BECOME SUCCESSFUL.

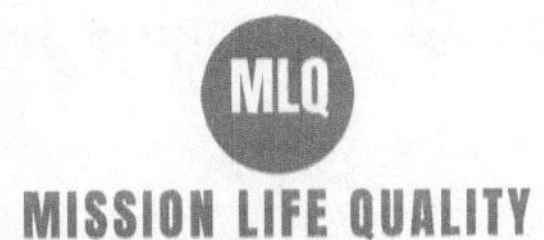

The information herein is offered for informational purposes solely and is universal as such. The presentation of the information is without a contract or any type of guarantee assurance.

The trademarks that are used are without any consent, and the publication of the trademark is without permission or backing by the trademark owner. All trademarks and brands within this book are for clarifying purposes only and are owned by the owners themselves, not affiliated with this document.

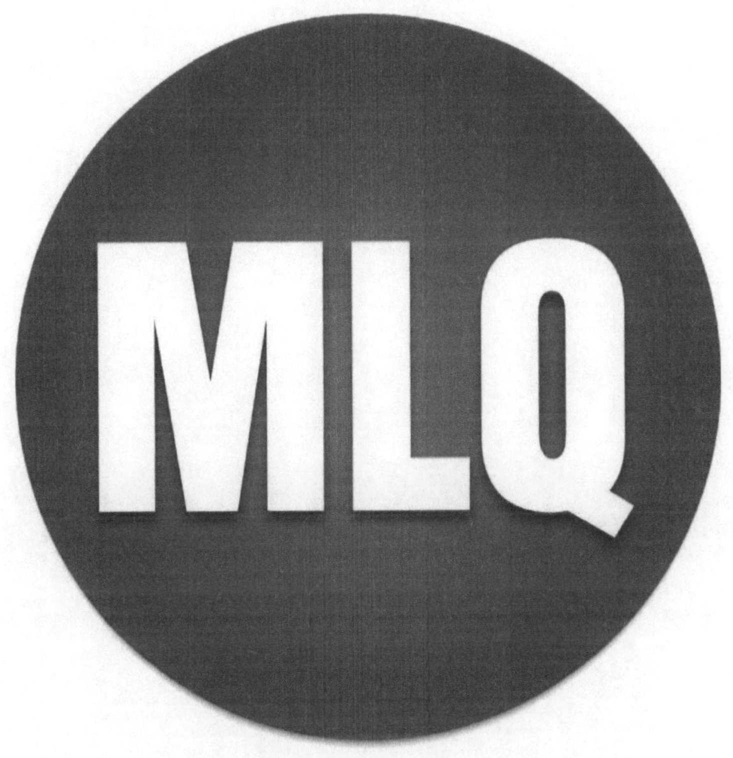

MISSION LIFE QUALITY

A brand devoted to the best quality of life, through a healthy nutrition, personal growth and much more.

TABLE OF CONTENTS

"In essence, if we want to direct our lives, we must take control of our consistent actions. It's not what we do once in a while that shapes our lives, but what we do consistently."

Tony Robbins

INTRODUCTION

Dear reader, it's with great pleasure that I welcome you to my book "Habits For Success". I thank you for purchasing "Habits For Success" and am excited to share my knowledge and experiences with you through this book. I hope this book can entertain you and add some value to your life.

"Habits For Success" is a book that teaches you all you need to know about good habits in your life. It will provide you with basic knowledge about the topic but will also go deeper into the specifics of habit formation. It will share with you many great habits that you can implement in your life not only to improve your productivity but also your quality of life. It will provide you with good advice to build up a morning routine that will set you up for success. On top of this, you will discover what unique habits successful people like Mark Zuckerberg or Elon Musk implemented in their life to become so successful.

The primary goal of this book is to show and enlighten the importance of taking control of your habits. Being able to implement good habits in your life and breaking bad ones means to be in control of your life. If you are in control of your habits you have the power to push your life to the next level and become the person you've always dreamed of. This book wants to show you in which ways you can benefit from good habits and how they can shape your life. It wants to provide you with valuable information not only regarding what habits to implement and why, but also how to effectively implement new habits in your life, improving your physical and mental well-being.

I want to thank you again for purchasing this book and hope the information I shared with you through this book will help you improve yourself.

I wish you a pleasant reading.

MY STORY

You'll never change your life until you change something you do daily. The secret of your success is found in your daily routine.

I have experienced many different habits in my life, both good ones, and bad ones, and I want to share with you the benefits I received and the lessons I learned from them. Samuel Johnson once said: "The chains of habits are too light to be felt, until they are too heavy to be broken." And I see that all the time, I see people that have self-destructive patterns, when they are in their 50s or 60s, and they can't change that because they are imprisoned by that.

In my personal experience, the right habits can help you increase your productivity exponentially. Life is habit. Or rather life is a succession of habits. It's all about finding the perfect mix, the perfect cocktail of habits, that best suits your personal needs and wishes. Not every habit is for everyone, some habits or rituals that are beneficial for certain people can be completely counterproductive for others. We are all different, and each of us has different needs and necessities.

Before trying to implement any new habit in your life, you need to know what you need to change about your life. Is it your productivity? Your attitude towards people? Or is it your diet? Only when you figure out what exactly you need to work on will you be able to find the habits that suit you. Once you've found the best combination for you, your productivity will soar. You will notice that you have much more energy and get much more done in a day. Having the right habits can really make the difference between living a healthy, happy, and productive life and living a stressful and painful life, which you are not in control of. Successful people are simply those with successful habits.

Implementing new habits and stick to them can be hard, most people give up after a couple of days, as they lack motivation and a sense of purpose. Implementing new habits in your life is hard, living a stressful life which you are not in control of is hard too. Eventually, it all comes down to choosing your "hard", choosing what kind of hardship you prefer to have in your life. This is the way you have to look at it, both options come with different hardships, and eventually, it's up to you to decide which ones you want to go through. Understand this thought-process and you will be successful in implementing whichever habit you want in your life.

Finding the perfect cocktail of habits has allowed me to benefit so incredibly much from them. I started getting so much more done every day. I started feeling so much better and healthier. It felt like my energy levels doubled. I was able to rush through all my to-do list faster and more productively than ever before. The trick to success is to choose the right habit and have just enough self-discipline to establish it. At the end of the day, I got way more done, while at the same time having a lot more extra time available that I could spend doing what I like. Being able to do what you like, knowing that you got everything done, gives you a true and unique sense of freedom. It's a never-ending process, you keep experimenting with new habits every month; it's like a journey, on which you broaden your knowledge every single step you take forward. Until the end of the journey, you keep learning and improving yourself.

HOW TO BUILD
GOOD HABITS
FOR LIFE

Habits are the small decisions you make and actions you perform every day. It is a routine of behavior that we subconsciously repeat regularly, which can be daily, weekly, or even monthly. We usually don't notice when we are exhibiting one of our habits. For instance, most of us barely notice when we brush our teeth in the morning. Habits are sometimes compulsory, we exhibit them unintentionally and cannot always control them fully. Approximately 43% of our daily behaviors are performed out of habit, which means that we're not completely aware of almost half of our daily behaviors. New behaviors can be learned automatically through the so-called habit formation process. We commonly talk about learning new good habits and break bad ones, but we have a really hard time doing so. Old habits are hard to break because the behavioral patterns, so the habits, that we repeat over a long period become imprinted in neural pathways, meaning our body exhibits them automatically. This also means that new habits can be formed through repetition over a longer period. Once you understand that habits can be changed, you have the freedom and the responsibility to remake them. Our life today is essentially the sum of our habits. How happy or unhappy are you? How successful or unsuccessful are you? What we repeatedly do ultimately forms the person we are, what we believe in, and shapes our personality. When you learn to transform your habits, you can transform your life.

Habits are not all the same, some habits may be so-called motor habits, meaning they refer to muscular activity and are related to our physical actions, such as running, walking, or doing exercise. Other habits are related to our mind, these are the so-called intellectual habits. Intellectual habits occur through a psychological process, such as observing, perceiving, or thinking, and do not involve physical action. Emotional habits instead, allow us to express our character and emotions. Being honest, hardworking, and being kind are some examples of emotional habits. These again don't describe a physical action and, as opposed to intellectual habits, are not as easily controllable. Emotions are influenced by our character, which we cannot control or change. You can only slightly alter your character purposefully. Normally your character changes over the course of time, through our growth and aging process, and is influenced by various external factors.

Habits form through a long process of repeating a certain behavior over the course of time until our subconscious mind eventually exhibits this behavior automatically. This process of habit formation can be slow, most of us need around two months to fully implement a new habit in our lives, but sometimes this process can take over six months.

To build a good habit, you need an excellent plan, motivation, and routine, otherwise, it is near to impossible to stick to your habits. I don't mean to frighten you or discourage you from pursuing this goal by any means, in fact, I'm trying to encourage you to take full control of your own life. Nevertheless, you need to understand that things don't come by themselves, while you sit back and relax, that's not how things work. As with anything else in your life, you need to work hard, to achieve it. You need to be aware that changing your daily routine, breaking bad habits, and replacing them with good ones takes a lot of physical effort and mental maturity. You need to have a plan and commit to it; you cannot skip days or procrastinate. If you make a commitment you need to stick with it, until you achieve your goal. Success is the sum of all the small efforts repeated day-by-day. It's about setting priorities; you need to create a sense of urgency in you, which will allow you to honor your commitment. Ultimately, it's a commitment you make to your future and to the version of you that you strive to become. Honor that commitment and you will be one step closer to that version of you, procrastinate and fail and you won't be making any progress.

The commitment you make to yourself to respect your new routine might seem tough to honor, but the reality is that it gets easier as you go. The first days are always the hardest, but as you get going everything smooths out and you will notice that it was far easier than expected. In fact, when you repeat a behavior for a long time, then it automatically becomes a habit. With a little bit of effort and commitment, it's easy to develop good habits in your life. It's just the starting phase that needs a lot of attention. You'll never change your life until you change something you do daily. The secret to success lays in your daily routine.

First of all, to implement new habits you need to keep in mind that every habit you have — good or bad — follows the same 3–step pattern: reminder (the trigger that initiates the behavior), routine (the behavior itself), and reward (the benefit you gain from doing the behavior). All of the 3 steps are equally important, and none of them should be skipped. The first stage, the reminder, or context cue can be a prior action, a specific time of the day, a location, or anything that triggers the habitual behavior. This could be anything that our mind associates with that habit, which automatically reminds us of our habit. A habit may initially be triggered by a goal, but over time the habit ends up slowly becoming automatic and we don't even need to think about it anymore. You need to find something that reminds you of your habit, something that triggers it. You can surely set reminders on your phone too, in fact, that is a very good possibility for certain habits. For others, you might have to come up with a different plan instead. Nevertheless, a strong commitment is already a good start.

The second stage, the behavior, is the actual habit that one exhibits. So, it's the action we perform as part of our habit, which can be exercising, reading a book, or eating breakfast. After you've been reminded of the action you need to take in order to implement your habit, you need to find a process or somewhat that makes you stick to it. Motivation is what gets you started, it's what gets the ball rolling. Habit instead, is what keeps you going in the long run. This could be a sense of guilt, you could think about how you are damaging yourself and your growth by not sticking to your plan, or it could be a photo above your bed, that triggers something in you. It is irrelevant what it is, it's paramount that you have some sort of guarantee that will withhold you from skipping that day and will make you exhibit that behavior.

Lastly, the reward is the benefit we gain from that very habit. A reward can be for instance a positive feeling. Sometimes the short-term reward that comes from exhibiting the habit isn't enough to keep one motivated, which is why intermittent rewards are particularly effective in promoting habit learning. For instance, when trying to start working out daily, you can tell yourself you will watch an episode of your favorite series if you first work out. This gives you a clearer purpose and stimulates you to keep up with your habit. The reward at first doesn't seem to play such an important role, but it does. Rewarding yourself for a specific behavior links pleasure to it and creates an emotional connection with the habit. That way it has a higher probability of repeating itself. Attach love to a new habit and you'll want to do it again. Some people might not think about a rewarding process after they've successfully completed their task, but you should keep this very well in mind. You need to always clearly visualize your whys. Why are you doing this? What is the benefit you are gaining from this? Where will this lead you? If you know the reason behind something though you need to get through, it will be much easier to get through it. If this isn't enough, you could, on top of this, reward yourself with something you come up with. You can for instance tell yourself that only if you achieve your goal, you'll get your favorite food for lunch, or you'll give yourself an extra 30 minutes to watch your favorite show. The bottom line is what we can control is our response to the stimuli and our actions, and that's where developing good habits matters. These three steps create a sort of "habit loop", which repeats itself every day. This helpful framework, once visualized and memorized, can further simplify the habit formation process and make it easier to stick to new habits so that you can improve your health, your work, and your life in general.

Once you've successfully stuck to your first good habit you are set to succeed and introduce many more productive habits in your routine. 'A good beginning is half done' is a promise. The first one is always the hardest, but once you started you will be positively surprised to see how your path smooths out and everything becomes easier. Making a good start does not mean that you should implement a bunch of new habits in your life at once; not at all. Instead, even though you will be very excited and motivated to start, you need to begin with small adjustments only. Do not start with too many habits! Most people try to achieve everything in a single day, which doesn't work, and they end up getting overwhelmed and give up. Instead of going for fixing everything in a small amount of time, it's better to focus on one habit at a time, making small, yet effective adjustments so that your mind can handle these gradual positive changes in a proper way Drop by drop is the water pot filled, and sooner than later you will have flipped your self-destructive patterns into highly effective routines.

Implementing a step-by-step approach to go through a process like this one is an efficient way of completing your tasks because step-by-step processes allow your mind to clearly visualize what needs to be done to achieve your goal, avoiding feeling overwhelmed. While trying to introduce new habits in your daily life you want to keep a positive mindset. Positive thinking not only helps you to overcome negative feelings but also enables you to deal with stress-related issues effectively. Being optimistic does not mean to ignore your commitments when you fail and simply go on with life, it means to react positively to the unpleasant events that you might encounter along your way. It becomes much easier for your mind to accept the new routine, if your thoughts are positive towards it. So, be positive and let go of the negative thoughts.

When talking about positivity, choosing a favorable environment can make the difference. Good habit formation also depends upon the encouraging atmosphere. For example, a student who wants to work hard will perform much better if he is surrounded by other hard-working students rather than lazy people who have no interest in studies. Such an environment will stimulate him to work harder and push himself to the next level, trying to keep up with the others.

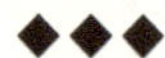

Once you've started to get used to your habit it becomes of paramount importance to keep up with it and strictly avoid any interruptions or postponements. It is essential to practice the new habit regularly; postponements or interruptions severely weaken your habit formation. Winning is not a sometime thing; it's an all-time thing. You don't win once in a while, you don't do things right once in a while, you do them right all the time, over and over again. Winning is a habit. Unfortunately, so is losing. If you start giving some lame excuses like a headache, or a mood and postpone your habit you will soon find yourself back where you started and all the progress you've previously made will be vane.

As we develop good habits various doubts might creep in. How long will it take? Can I really make it? Will I have enough discipline to keep up with it? I want you to remember one thing, may this be the only thing you remember out of the entire book, but make sure to remember it:

"Self-doubt kills more dreams than failure ever will".

Don't strive for an overnight life-change, you need to keep in mind that this is a long-term process that requires consistent work and dedication, thus focus on the 1% improvement. A 1% daily improvement will get you farther than you might expect. People tend to overestimate what they can do in one day, but underestimate what they can do in a whole year. Having one amazing training session will not make an athlete fit, but four consistent training sessions per week over an entire year definitely will. It's important to remember that we're focusing on consistent improvements over a long period of time, not instant gains. Habits compounded over multiple weeks, months and years will yield massive results and that's all that matters. It's always possible to find a 1% improvement, so keep striving to be a bit better than you were yesterday and eventually you'll get there. Every great accomplishment starts with the simple decision to try.

MORNING RITUALS

When you arise in the morning, think of what a precious privilege it is to be alive, to breathe, to think, to enjoy, to love. Do not waste the opportunity to make something out of your life. The morning is the most valuable time of the day, it can set the tone for your entire day. The right morning routine can make the difference between a super-productive day or a sluggish one. Yet many people take their mornings for granted, they sleep in, don't have a healthy breakfast, and have to rush to make it in time to work or whatever other appointments, starting their day with a big dose of stress and tiredness. These self-destructive habits shape all of your mornings and influence your whole day. The time between waking up and getting to work is not a blur. The tone of our mornings has a powerful ripple effect on our mood, happiness, and focus for the rest of the day. It becomes a cycle: wake up stressed, spend the rest of the day feeling that way, go to sleep feeling anxious, and repeat.

Each morning we are born again. What we do today is what matters most. A year from now, you may wish you had started today.

A good morning routine provides a way to feel accomplished and reach new levels of success. It allows you to boost your productivity and motivation exponentially, allowing you to be much more effective and efficient. This is why many highly successful people — from Barack Obama to Oprah, Bill Gates, and Elon Musk — have crafted morning rituals that maximize their energy, productivity, and creativity all day long.

But what makes a good routine? I don't believe there exists anything like "the perfect morning routine", as for everyone there is a specific routine that works best. Everyone has different needs and priorities, which means that everyone needs to find the right routine for themselves. You need to create your personal morning ritual: Maybe you like to go for a run or maybe you enjoy meditating and find your peace of mind. Whatever it is that boosts your energy and mood, kickstart your day with that cocktail of habits. Establishing a meaningful morning ritual will help you start your day on a much more positive and productive note. Structure your day in advance giving yourself enough time to go through your routine, you do not want to rush through your mornings. This will without any doubt eliminate stress, mental fatigue, and enhance your productivity. You will not come up with the perfect routine by googling it and picking out a couple of habits. Building up an effective morning routine takes time, you will need to start with certain habits and then, as you go, eliminate the ones you don't benefit enough from and introduce new ones until you feel you found the sweet-spot.

The prerogative to a successful morning routine is planning. Planning is the first and most important step in this context. If you fail to plan, you are planning to fail. You want to put down a plan for your day and for your week in advance. I highly recommend before going to bed to take pen and paper and write down your commitments and goals for the next day, whether it's something to achieve in business, or in life, or a deadline you need to meet. While long-term goals are what we tend to focus on, it's the daily goals that we set that allow us to create short-term milestones that are integral to our success. Long-term goals usually seem overwhelming when you look at them, but by implementing a daily goal-setting strategy, you can overcome some of the enormity associated with achieving big things in life by focusing on the day by day short-term scenarios.

While structuring your plan, think in time-blocking, not in minute by minute. You want to be as specific as possible concerning the activities and their duration. You want to plan enough time for each of your activities, making sure to add short five-minute-breaks here and there. When setting your goals for the day, you don't want to set goals that are unrealistic, or that you know you will not be able to achieve. Instead, you need to set realistic and achievable goals, that you can achieve if you work hard enough. You'll get more done and will be less stressed than if you jump into your day without a plan. The truth is, we're all working towards some big achievement that matters to us. Nevertheless, it's your daily goals that help you stay on your path and allow you to develop short-term goals that are essential for your success, because if you don't know where you are going, you will probably end up somewhere else.

Setting your goals is one thing, achieving them is another. When working towards a goal you want to put yourself in a condition that allows you to be as productive and as efficient as possible. It is scientifically proven that people are much more effective and focused during the early morning hours than they are during the rest of the day. The early morning hours are a time for peaceful reflection and ample productivity, when the world is still and asleep, allowing you to focus wholeheartedly on your goals. The key to success is to have lunch at the same time that most people have breakfast. Anyone who is serious about success knows that it's important to wake up early. Some people dream of success, while others get up every morning and make it happen. Waking up as early as 5:00 a.m. is one of the most popular morning routines to increase the own productivity. A 2008 study found that early risers procrastinated not nearly as much as people who get up late. It's not a surprise, as in the morning people don't have nearly any distractions and can thus work in a quiet and distraction-free environment to complete their tasks. Waking up early is not only beneficial to your productivity and efficiency, but it's also a good way to relieve stress. Let's say you have to be out of the door by 8:00 a.m. and you don't get out of bed until 7:30 a.m., then you will have to rush through your morning routine: showering, brushing your teeth, maybe grab something to eat on your way, and most likely you will end up forgetting something. If instead, you woke up at 6:00 a.m. you would have two hours to get ready. You would have enough time to go through a decent morning routine, have a great breakfast, brush your teeth, watch the news and maybe shower or do whatever else you like to do in the morning. You would have time not only to get ready but also to catch up on emails or work on a project. Former President Barack Obama for instance would always start his day in the White House two hours before his first scheduled meeting, which meant he got up as early as 5:00 a.m., which allowed him to prioritize exercise, an activity he never missed. Such a routine would make your mornings less stressful, which in turn, would make your days less stressful and you would be happier and calmer. A study conducted by the Roehampton University in London found that morning people tend to be healthier and happier as well as having lower body mass indexes. I cannot overemphasize the importance of getting up early enough, even if you're not a morning person, you need to stick to this habit. Lose an hour in the morning, and you will spend the rest of the day looking for it. If you are struggling, you can use incremental changes in your daily routine to start waking up earlier. A great way to do this is by setting your alarm back by 15 minutes every week until you can wake up at least two hours earlier than you're waking up now. A progressive approach allows your body more time to get used to the new routine, making it a very effective way to approach this habit.

A great thing to do right after you jump out of bed is making your bed. Making your bed gives you a sense of accomplishment helping you to start the day in the right way. By making your bed you successfully completed your first task of the day. It is a great way to practice self-discipline as it teaches you to follow your inner voice. You learn not to procrastinate or give up, but rather get done what needs to be done. It's a way of training your body to do what you want it to do, instead of listening to your feelings of tiredness and sleepiness.

As you got out of bed you want to start your early morning in the best possible way: with a healthy and energizing breakfast. Breakfast is the most important meal of the day, yet over 30 million Americans skip breakfast every day. Eating a healthy breakfast can make a remarkable difference in your day. Your body needs a certain amount of food on regular intervals to function properly. By skipping breakfast, you end up fasting until lunch. Since the last time you had a proper meal was the evening before, you effectively fasted for over 16 hours. How can this be healthy for your body? In order to be successful in what you do and be able to work at your 100% first of all you need to make sure your body is at its 100%. To get your body to its 100% it needs enough sleep and enough healthy food. Not feeding your body and expecting it to take you through your workday, is like expecting your car to take you from the East Coast to the West Coast with an empty tank. It simply does not work. And if we want to be precise, you want to fuel your car with the best fuel, the purest and the most performing one. So, in the same way as your car, you want to feed your body with vitamins, proteins, and carbs. There is a ton of information out there about nutrition, do not ignore it, take advantage of it. Learn what to fuel your body with, in order to get the best out of it. This habit certainly requires some planning, but if you give yourself enough time in the morning to enjoy an energizing breakfast, nothing will stop you throughout the day.

While eating breakfast most of us enjoy to turn on the TV and listen to the latest news. I would argue that this indeed is not the best way to start your day. Listening to the news or reading the newspaper first thing in the morning is or can be counterproductive, as it shifts the focus away from yourself and your self-motivation for the day and shifts it towards external events. Your focus determines your reality. Make yourself a priority. At the end of the day, you are your longest and most important commitment. Watching the news is important indeed, I am not trying to say the opposite. Nevertheless, consider if it truly is the information you want to feed your brain with in the morning. I think you should avoid watching the news at the start of your day, as your focus needs to be on yourself first of all, mentally preparing for your day. Only throughout your day, or better, at the end of the day, you should catch up on the news.

Your mind and your body are not separate, what affects one, affects the other. This is why as you try to develop good habits for your mind, you should develop some good habits for your body as well. Eating a healthy breakfast, is certainly a good start, but, in addition to that, taking a cold shower would be even more beneficial for your body. Taking a cold shower not only helps to calm itchy skin, but it also helps reducing muscle soreness after having worked out. The most important benefit from taking a cold shower, and the main reason many experts recommend it, is because it increases your blood circulation. Coldwater, as it hits your body, constricts circulation on the surface of your body. This causes blood in your deeper tissues to circulate at faster rates to maintain an ideal body temperature. In that sense, a hot shower instead, has the opposite effect for someone with hypertension or a cardiovascular disease. Exposure to cold temperatures, on the other hand, triggers the circulatory system to reduce inflammation and to a certain extent, helps prevent a cardiovascular disease. And if on top of that, you need to get an adrenaline boost and wake up quickly, you definitely want to take that cold shower as soon as you step out of bed. Studies showed how taking regular cold showers can help with weight loss, as certain cells of our body burn fat to generate heat, but I would argue how much a cold shower realistically benefits you in this way. Wrapping up, a cold shower that increases your air intake and your heart rate, and boosts your alertness, definitely helps you start your day in a better way. If you don't feel comfortable with taking a cold shower in the morning, you should start by washing your face with cold water in the morning and after two weeks you try to take a cold shower in the morning.

Depending on how serious you are on this morning routine, you may want to consider the below and take your morning routine to a whole new level. You have most likely already heard, at least once, of morning meditation and its benefits. Mindful meditation early in the morning helps you place yourself in the present moment. It enables you to be mindful of challenging situations during the day. Meditation allows you to be in tune with your inner universe and dissolves the invisible walls that unawareness has built. Different stressors may trigger as you go through the day, but some good meditation can help you remain calm before taking on the challenges. Personally, it's helped me a lot to control my emotions. Meditation calms me down and helps me having better control over my reactions to outer stimuli. Meditation is a good habit to have if you want to be connected to what is significant in your life.
Another benefit of meditation is the positive emotions like empathy and kindness it promotes. The deep state of flow that meditation induces builds social connectedness and makes us more affectionate and friendly as a person. Quiet the mind and the soul will speak. From a productivity standpoint meditation improves the brain's problem-

solving and decision-making capabilities, which can bring a desirable shift in your professional life. On top of this meditation is known to be a great stress reliever and boosts your well-being and happiness in general. Correct your mind and the rest of your life will fall into place. The great thing about meditation is that it's very easily accessible and everyone can meditate for how long and in what way they want. You can go on a walk and meditate in the woods, or you can just sit on the floor of your bedroom, close your eyes and meditate for 20 minutes. There are a lot of resources out there and thousands of apps you can download on your phone to take your meditation to an even deeper level. Meditation is a very broad subject, there are a lot of different ways to meditate and a lot of reasons to do so.

BODY AND WELL-BEING

"Fall in love with taking care of your body"

The greatest wealth is health. Your body is the most valuable possession of yours. Your body is a part of you, it's your engine, it's what keeps you going. Your body is what allows you to do what you love; it gives you the mobility and strength you need to reach your goals. Your body is a wonderful tool you have, which has unlimited potential. Taking care of your body and making sure you always put it in a condition to express its capabilities and potential at its fullest, should be your primary concern. Yet, so many people don't give enough value to their bodies, the backbone of their life. Too many people do not give it the necessary stimuli and resources it needs. A body not taken care of is like a machine that doesn't receive any maintenance. It will be cheaper and less stressful to operate at first, that is for sure, but at some point, that machine will stop functioning and will break. Our body needs to be maintained and provided with what it needs. If not maintained, health problems will soon arise. Health problems, even minor ones, can interfere with other aspects of your life. Even relatively minor health issues such as a headache, or indigestion take a toll on your happiness and stress levels. Poor health habits add substantial stress to your life and also play a role in how well you can cope with it. If you think you have no time for healthy eating, you will sooner or later have to find time for illness. Health problems can make daily tasks more challenging, and even jeopardize your ability to earn a living. One way to improve your health and feel better is to commit to healthier habits, which will definitely, I assure you, pay off in the long run. But what exactly does our body need? How can we improve our health and well-being? There are three main things your body needs to be provided with: enough rest and sleep, healthy nutrition, and a lot of exercise, all of which are necessities, not luxuries.

"You are what you eat", is what most nutritionists will tell you when discussing the importance of your nutrition. It's become a bit of a cliché recently, nevertheless, its truthfulness is not up for discussion. Our brains need the right food to perform at their best. The food we eat can be either the best medicine or the worst form of poison. Never go to work with an empty stomach, it will be detrimental to your performance. People need to train themselves to eat a balanced and healthy diet. It's important to learn this already at a young age, as we tend to carry the habits we learn when we are young forward with us for most of our lives. We don't value health until sickness comes. Learning what to introduce in your body now can avoid many health issues down the road.

We shall take care of our body, it's the only place we have to live in. Obesity, high cholesterol levels, high blood pressure, and diabetes are all common problems in our modern lives and are usually a direct result of poor diets. When your diet is wrong, medicine is of no use. When your diet is correct, medicine is of no need. Modern diets usually contain too many processed foods that are high in fats, sugar, and salt. A more balanced diet should include more fresh fruit and vegetables, the vitamins of which will strongly improve your and immune system. Many scientists now argue that portion control and diet balancing are two of the most important aspects of eating healthy. Perhaps the best approach is to make sure that you eat a little bit of everything. Your goal is to get enough of each essential building block of diet. You want to have a balance between fats, carbs, and proteins, avoiding an overdose of any of these. It's not about looking better in your jeans; not at all. It's about boosting your energy levels and keeping your system running smoothly. This is because what you eat can not only impact your short-term condition but also your long-term health. A healthy outside starts from the inside. Hunger can make you more emotionally reactive to stressors, leaving you irritable or even angry in the face of minor daily annoyances. Being smart about what you eat can be a stress management tool as well as a health preserver. Eating foods that are rich in nutrients can also boost your energy levels. In order to get those nutrients, you want to make sure that your healthy diet includes not only fruit and vegetables but also whole grains and low-fat dairy products, as well as lean meats.

Sometimes you might not have the time to prepare a healthy meal, or you might not have thought about something healthy to make. This is why planning your meals in advance is really important. Doing this in the morning, or the day before will save you from last-minute unhealthy food choices when you are having a bad day. You might want to plan it even more in advance so that you can properly plan what groceries to buy and what to prepare. It might not seem such a relevant thing to do, but it really does make the difference. When you plan your meals you typically tend to choose the healthier option, whereas when you need to choose your meal last-minute you are more prone to give in to unhealthy options, which you cannot resist. So, if you never preplan your meals you are very likely to have a much unhealthier diet. You really want to avoid that, as a healthy diet is 50% of the work towards a healthy, in-shape body.

The remaining 50% of the work towards a healthy body is exercise. Exercise is not a punishment for what you ate, it's a celebration of what your body can do. Doing sports regularly is the best, most beneficial habit for you and your life. Every day is another chance to get stronger, to eat better, to live healthier, and to be the best version of yourself. Practicing sports daily doesn't have to be heavy weightlifting or running a marathon. Lightly strenuous activities are good enough to oxygenate your blood and boost the endorphins in your body. The pain you feel while exercising, will be the strength you feel in the future. Doing sports will make you feel so much better, it is a proven stress reliever and it helps you restore your motivation and energies if you are studying or working very hard. Going out in the open air for a run clears your mind and helps you be more emotionally sound. Exercise releases dopamine, oxytocin, and serotonin into your body, inducing a euphoric feeling.

Exercise is the most underutilized antidepressant. Exercise elevates mood by boosting the production of endorphins, hormones that act as natural anti-depressants. How often do you tell yourself that you do not have time for exercising? Stop pretending you do not have time. In life it's all about priorities, you can make time for something if you prioritize it over your other activities. It all comes down to the importance you give to your body and your health, nothing should have priority over your own health, not even your job. Most successful people exercise every day, not only to keep physically in shape but also to stimulate their creativity and cognitive skills. Thus, if you don't have time to exercise, your priorities need to change. Even just a 15-minute-exercise session is better than nothing. The only bad workout is the one that didn't happen. Jack Dorsey, the CEO of Twitter, said: "I wake up every day by 5:00, meditate for thirty minutes, seven-minute workout times three, make coffee, and check-in." He said it gives him a steady-state that empowers him to be more productive.

Some people find ways, others find excuses. A very efficient way of doing exercise is trying to implement it in your daily schedule. For instance, you could walk or ride a bike to work instead of driving your car, if possible. Or you could use the stairs instead of the elevator. Not using the elevator is a commonly known habit and its benefits are widely known too. Not taking the elevator can make you walk more than 10,000 extra steps every day. A very interesting study provided shocking results of how many steps people in different countries take daily. Americans, on average, take little over 5,000 steps a day. Australians and Swiss people instead, take a whopping 9,700 steps per day, and the Japanese take around 7,200 steps per day. Even still, this single habit is a great way to resolve our sedentary ways. Park further from the office or take the stairs when you can to boost your daily steps.

We're used to living a very stressful and busy life, which our body can sometimes not keep up with. That's why it can sometimes be a great help to take supplements, especially if our diet is lacking certain nutrients. As a culture, we often lack the necessary vitamins and minerals from our food intake. Processed and refined sugars, carbohydrates, and other foods that a staple of the American diet, help to exacerbate this problem. You need to find a good set of vitamins and minerals that you can take on a daily basis. It's easy to ignore this healthy habit, but the feeling after weeks and months of taking supplements regularly is incredible. That impact can help us improve other areas of our lives by providing mental, emotional, and physical improvements.

Not all people are comfortable with taking supplements, if you are a more natural-oriented person, there are various natural treatments as well. Drinking water with lemon is a good example. Yes, in fact, this habit has monumental health benefits. Lemons are a natural source of Vitamin C, but also possess other health benefits, which help with your digestion, boost your immune system and cleanse and rehydrate your body. According to the USDA, one lemon has between 30-45 g of Vitamin C, which is 30-40% of the recommended daily intake. A big glass of water with lemon every day will substantially help your body grow healthier. Even just water itself is a great method to flush any toxins from your system. Another great way to improve your nutrition is by eliminating all kinds of sodas and drinks high in carbohydrates, such as cokes and energy drinks. You don't notice it, because you don't see it, but the amount of sugar that you introduce in your body with those drinks is impressive. If you had to eat all that plain sugar without the drink, you would never be able to. Our nutrition is the most powerful drug available, it has the power to cause or cure most diseases. Avoiding sodas will also aid with weight loss, inflammations, and your overall body energy.

As we previously discussed, the three main things your body requires are: a healthy diet, a lot of exercise, and last but not least enough rest and sleep. Sleep is the golden chain that binds our health and our body together. Sleep is what most of us lack nowadays due to our extremely busy schedules. Cutting back on sleep in order to get more done in a day is a very bad strategy. When your body lacks sleep it cannot perform, your brain will not be able to absorb any new information, and it will have a hard time focusing. Getting enough sleep helps you deal with negativity better, while also keeping you healthy. Research has found that getting plenty of sleep strengthens your immune system. The ideal strategy to get more sleep would be, not to wake up later, but to go to bed earlier, in order to get at least eight hours of sleep. Early sleep and early wake up makes you healthy and makes you grow. Going to bed earlier allows you to get enough sleep, while still being able to get up early and take advantage of the early morning hours to be productive. Eight hours a day of sleep is what an average person needs. Finding that delicate balance might be difficult, especially if your private life comes in between. However, if you care enough about your physical well-being, along with your future success, you'll focus on a minimum of eight hours of uninterrupted sleep every night. Remember that muscles are torn in the gym, fed in the kitchen, and built in bed. If you have trouble falling asleep, be wary not to drink coffee or alcohol too close to your bedtime. Eating dinner earlier can also help you falling asleep easier, as after you eat, your body needs various hours, depending on the meal, to digest the food you've just eaten, and if you go to bed while still having to digest you will have a tough time falling asleep. Nicotine, too much sugar, or other toxins are also detrimental to your ability to go to bed at a reasonable time.

You can't enjoy wealth if you're not in good health. Constant pains and aches have a detrimental effect on your health and happiness. More and more people, especially men nowadays have to cope with back pain or other pains. The causes for such pains can vary and can sometimes be serious too, but keeping a good posture is certainly a good first step. A good posture is not about standing up straight to look at your best on your social media. It is a milestone for your long-term health. Making sure you hold your body the right way will prevent pain, injuries, and other major health concern as you get older.

We generally tend to differentiate between dynamic and static postures. The first one being how you hold yourself when you are moving, walking, running, etc.; and the latter one being how you hold yourself when you are standing still, sitting, sleeping, etc. The main cause of severe back pain is how people hold their body when lifting heavyweights. See, the problem is that most people, when lifting weights, primarily use their back's strength, both to lift the weight, as well as to carry it. Lifting weights in this way is suicidal for your spine, it severely damages it. Instead of using your back, you should instead take advantage of your legs' strength. When you are lifting a heavyweight from the ground, instead of bending your back, you should bend your legs, while keeping your back straight up, and when you are lifting the weight, use your legs' muscles to get up. In this way your spine won't be under pressure, thus preventing any damage to it.

Since most of us spend various hours sitting, whether it's at work, at school, or at home, an inappropriate static posture takes a toll on your health. The key to the best posture is the position of your spine. Your spine is not straight, it has a wavy shape, with three natural curves: at your neck, mid-back, and low back. The ideal posture should maintain these natural curves, without increasing or decreasing them. When you are sitting for a longer time, it's important to make sure you keep a balanced posture. Your body should form a 90-degree angle at your hips, and so should your legs at your knees. You can easily check this by making sure your head is directly above your shoulders, not bent forwards, or backwards. Your shoulder should be aligned with your hips, both laterally, to prevent misalignments of the musculoskeletal system, which could result in scoliosis, as well as longitudinally, to maintain the spine's natural curves. These little details will allow you to avoid major neck, shoulder, and back pain, as well as preserve your joints' movement ability. On top of this always make sure that your work surfaces are at a comfortable height, that your feet always touch the ground, and that your elbows are kept close to your body. Avoid crossing your legs and wearing heeled shoes and gently stretch your muscles every now and then.

Checking your posture is more important than most people think it is. We usually don't even notice how bad our posture is when we sit in front of the computer or lay on the couch. Keeping a healthy posture will help make the difference in your 50s and 60s when your back is going to give you a hard time. A good piece of advice to improve your posture is to set a timer to check your posture every ten to fifteen minutes, you'll notice big improvements. I bet you just checked your posture this very moment.

A great habit I found, is to get some natural light when working on my computer at home. Even if you are very busy with work, just take your laptop and go work outside in the sun for at least an hour. Getting natural light every day is extremely beneficial for our skin and our mood. As the sun's rays touch our skin, they stimulate our body to release dopamine, a substance that makes us feel happy. The sun is furthermore a great source of Vitamin D, which regulates the amount of calcium and phosphate in the body. Vitamin D improves your mood, cognition, and pain tolerance. These nutrients are needed to keep bones, teeth, and muscles healthy. A lack of vitamin D leads to bone deformities such as rickets in children, and osteomalacia in adults, which causes bone pain.

Taking care of your body also means taking care of your hygiene. Habits like brushing your teeth twice a day and washing your hands regularly not only contribute to your health but also lead to building routines, which get you used to the process of implementing habits. Good hygiene is valuable for your body in general and makes you feel great. Good hygiene makes you look better too, allowing you to make a positive first impression. If you learn to have good hygiene you will learn to take care of your body and its needs. You can improve your hygiene by scraping your tongue. The clearest and most obvious benefit of tongue scraping is to get rid of the stinky breath you have when you get out of bed. If you want, you can take it a step further a scrub your tongue in the evening too. Scrubbing your tongue effectively removes bacteria, fungi, dead cells, and toxins from your mouth. Another way to get rid of your mouth bacteria is by rinsing your mouth with mouthwash. Mouthwash, besides getting rid of your bad breath also helps with tooth decay. The American Dental Association recommends using mouthwashes that contain cetylpyridinium chloride, which removes your bad breath, chlorhexidine, and essential oils, which can be used to control plaque and gingivitis, fluoride, which prevents tooth decay, and peroxide, which is present in whitening mouthwashes.

MIND AND PRODUCTIVITY

"The body achieves what the mind believes."

You have power over your mind, not over outside events. Realize this, and you will find strength. The mind is the most powerful tool you have. Its capabilities are endless, and its potential is unimaginable. Our brain is the most complex organ of ours, and as of 2020 we still haven't been able to fully comprehend how it works and what this magnificent organ is capable of. Our brain is arguably the most important part of our body. It controls and coordinates all our actions and reactions and allows us to think, feel, and remember. Our thoughts, perceptions, emotions, reasoning processes, and intelligence are all products of our brain. They are what makes up our mind. Develop a strong mind and you will lead a strong life. Our mind is very flexible and can be improved, stimulated, and developed in many different ways. Some of which depend on our behavior, yes because, we can in certain ways stimulate our mind and train it so that it develops further. Train your mind to be stronger than your emotions, otherwise your emotions will ruin you. Our productivity, however, depends directly from our mind, from our work ethic and from the ability of our mind to work hard. We want to put ourselves in a condition that allows us, or better, stimulates us to be as productive as we can.

A great way to kickstart your day on a productive and proficient note is to write your own daily journal. Yes, writing a journal, depending on the variation, can help you visualize what is going through your mind, it helps you process your thoughts and worries, making you feel better. Writing a journal is also a great way to find self-motivation to work towards a goal. Journaling is like whispering to the own self and listening at the same time. It is very effective in giving you an overview of all that you are planning to work on and what you want to achieve, and at the same time makes you aware of your progress. A journal is an exceptional way to manage your mental health, especially if you are going through a hard time. Journaling helps us stop, take a step back, and think about ourselves. You might find it helpful to write down all your thoughts and concerns in your journal, it allows you to open yourself up, giving you a feeling of freedom and relief. Journal writing is a journey to your interior universe.

There are several variations of journaling. You can write a paragraph based on what you're thinking, or simply write down your main thoughts and moods in point form. A journal can serve many different purposes as well, it can be used to cope with mental hardships, but also to boost your productivity and reduce your stress. In order to journal you need to set aside a few minutes every day to write. I've found the most ideal time to do this to be in the evening before going to bed. Another way to approach this is to have pen and paper with you at all times so that when something goes through your mind you can put it down on paper right away. Do not overthink this, you do not want to follow a strict structure and a fixed topic, you want this to be a place where your mind can completely open without any boundaries. It's important to write about whatever you feel the need to write about. Because in your journal you do not just express yourself more openly than you would to any other person: you create yourself!

One great way of journaling is to start a dream journal. Dreams are the window into our subconscious mind. If you are someone who remembers your dreams nearly every day, writing them down can bring awareness to some of your deeper thoughts, fears, and emotions. Writing down your dreams, if you are someone who happens to dream often, is a great way to analyze your mind. It allows you to visualize your dreams over a longer period of time and maybe you can recognize a certain pattern or a certain recurrent dream. Analyzing and understanding your dreams can help you understand your mind and learn what your thoughts, goals, fears, or stressors are.

Another interesting way of journaling is by writing down affirmations. Any affirmations about yourself, about your situation, about something you want to reach on a personal level, or a material goal you want to achieve, everything you feel the need to say can be written down. This process greatly boosts your self-esteem and helps you work towards your goals. Our greatest weapon against stress is our ability to choose one thought over another. Since affirmations can produce such positive results, they are worth experimenting with.

Not everyone might be passionate about writing a journal, as they might not appreciate the writing process of it. What I started doing, which in my opinion is a great way to visualize your progress in life is to record vlogs. You can approach this in various ways, rather than recording daily 30-second-videos, I prefer to record a long video every bunch of months where I record myself talking about my current situation in life and what my plans and goals for the future are. This habit helped me greatly, especially during rainy days, when I would just go back to those vlogs, and could clearly see the progress I've made from one video to the other, boosting my mood. You will be impressed by your growth from one video to the next one, which in turn will boost your motivation and self-confidence greatly. You can talk about whatever you want, whatever is relevant to you and your life, which can be your career or your relationship, or something completely different. Another approach is to record daily 1-minute videos. Personally, I am not a fan of this approach, since I think the effort for it obscures the actual benefits. Moreover, you can barely notice the progress you make between the videos. Nevertheless, it can still be beneficial if you just need to talk and open yourself up in order to get a better overview of what you need to focus on in the next days. You can talk about what's happening in your life, what you're grateful for, what you're thinking about, or simply choose a random speech topic. Both of these approaches are an excellent way to become a better speaker by watching your videos and bringing awareness to your pacing, how you articulate your thoughts, or how often you use filler words like 'um', 'so', or 'and' at the start of a sentence.

Talking about your speaking skills, a great way to practice your speaking skills is through storytelling. In business and in life, storytelling is an essential tool. Good storytelling skills can make the difference between a successful business, with many clients and investors, and a struggling business that fails to convince its audience and struggles to deliver any value to its customers. The same applies to you: if you have good storytelling skills you will be able to convince other people, you will be able to win discussions and gain credibility, and your career will positively benefit from this skill as well. Luckily, this is a skill that can easily be learned through practice. Writing, video logs or recording yourself are all good ways to practice storytelling. Get yourself in front of a camera and start recording yourself talking about a certain topic. This habit can result in creating a YouTube channel, which is a great way to influence big audiences. Make your way up until you end up talking in front of hundreds of people in real life and influencing the lives of thousands. If you make it your goal to add as much value as possible to as many people as possible, you'll never have to worry about success, because what you do for yourself alone dies with you, but what you do for others is never going to be forgotten.

> *"Whenever you give, it's always going to come back. Just give! The rewards will be greater than you can ever imagine."*
>
> *Tony Robbins*

Learning new skills and increasing our own knowledge is something all of us should strive for every day. Knowledge is power. The best life-investment you can make is to invest in your knowledge. An investment in knowledge always pays the best interest. Our knowledge is what makes us who we are, it shapes our believes and allows us to have an opinion. Our knowledge will determine whether we will succeed in life or not. I cannot overemphasize how important it is to further your knowledge. The best way to do so is through books. Reading books is a life-changing habit, the right book can revolutionize your life completely. Reading daily is one of the best habits, and long-term investments you can make. Reading can help you uncover new worlds, ideas, or ways of doing things that you might not have known about before. It's also a great way to educate yourself or entertain yourself at any given moment. It doesn't even really matter what you read, whether it's the newspaper, a novel, a non-fiction book, or anything else, you just need to find something you like to read. I would personally recommend choosing a book of your liking and read a couple of pages every day. You can decide when you want to read, nevertheless, I would not recommend reading right before going to bed, as you will be too tired, and your brain will have a hard time to process new information.

If you do not want to read paper books, you can try with kindle eBooks or audiobooks. Audiobooks are a great alternative to reading books and, in opposition to books, can be taken everywhere and listened to whenever. You can easily listen to an audiobook while you go for a walk, or while you are cooking. You can absorb content from books without even having to read them. This advantage of audiobooks will allow you to go through a book much faster and efficiently. If you are a fast learner, I would suggest you slowly increase the speed up to 1.5x or even 2x, this way you can absorb more information in a shorter timespan!

Listening to podcasts is another very good habit that you can add to your routine. There are so many options for excellent audio content to learn from and be inspired by. If you listen to a lot of music every day, then for one week, just one week, replace the music with podcasts of your liking. You will discover how beneficial it is to your mind, and how much you learn every day. Give it a week, and you won't stop listening to podcasts anymore. In the same way as an audiobook, podcasts allow you to do something else while you are listening to them, like getting ready, driving, or cleaning up, which allows you to maximize your time and get the most out of your days.

◆◆◆

When you discover a new topic that you are interested in and want to learn more about it, having good study habits might come in handy. Studying effectively is a valuable skill. Never regard study as a duty, but as the enviable opportunity to learn. People that live life to the fullest are lifelong learners. They never stop trying new things out and feeding their brain with new knowledge. In order to gather as much knowledge as you can, you need an effective and efficient method. Learning how to study and acquire the knowledge to succeed doesn't just occur naturally. It needs to be taught. Take a study skills course or ask others for tips on improving your study habits.

First of all, when trying to study it's of paramount importance that you learn to single-task. Multitasking is extremely unproductive, only 2% of people in the world can multitask successfully. Constantly juggling between tasks limits your focus, contributes to mental clutter, and makes it difficult for your brain to filter out irrelevant information. Stanford University found out that heavy multitasking lowers efficiency and impairs your cognitive control. Do not work on two different tasks contemporarily, rather come up with a plan and go through each of your tasks one by one. The absolute worst and most detrimental thing for your productivity is multitasking with your phone. It's been scientifically proven that multitasking with your phone reduces your productivity more than smoking marijuana. Multitasking with electronic media reduces a person's IQ by a staggering 10 points, more than twice the impact of smoking marijuana! The problem with multitasking with your phone is that you get easily distracted and lose awareness of time.

Most of our lack of productivity comes from a lack of concentrated work. Distractions destroy action. If it's not moving you towards your purpose, leave it be. There will always be distractions if you allow them. This is why you want to get rid of all the distractions around you, starting with your phone. Your phone is the biggest distraction; thus, you need to turn off your phone until you are completely done with your work. When you are done with a task you can allow yourself a five-minute-break and check your phone. When you need to work on something, create a comfortable environment around you that allows you to work in peace without being interrupted. Being 100% focused will allow you to finish your work so much faster and proficiently. A recent study conducted by the University of Chicago quite interestingly showed the effect smartphones have on the students' abilities. In the experiment, students were divided into two separate groups. One group was asked to leave their phones in a different room, while the other group was asked to silence their phones and leave them face down on their desk. The results were quite remarkable, in fact, the group asked to leave their phones in a different room performed noticeably better than the other group. Moreover, the study discovered that the distraction caused by smartphones happens on an unconscious level as well, as the majority of students said they weren't even thinking about their phones during the entire experiment. This is a quite surprising result and means that our phones reduce our ability to focus merely by being in the same room.

Most of us don't even notice how much time we spend on our phones daily. Unfortunately for us most apps and websites are programmed to be as addictive as possible, keeping us on the phone for hours. Apple thankfully introduced a screen-time tracker on its phones, which allows you to see how much time you spend daily or weekly on your phone and how you spend that time, meaning what apps you use more frequently. Most of you would be surprised by how much time you spend on your phone every day. I was shocked when I found out I occasionally spent over 8 or 9 hours a day on my phone. When we are on our phones, we lose awareness of time and waste precious hours on irrelevant things. Going for a social media detox can be very beneficial to you and your life, it can show you how bad you are investing your time. Research has shown that the more time you spend on social media, the more likely you are to develop depression. Take time to cut back on social media to reduce stress and mental clutter. Switch off your phone and laptop for a few hours every day to improve your mood and reconnect with the world around you. Find another habit or occupation that allows you to spend more hours off of your phone. I found riding a dirt-bike a thrilling and fun way of getting off of my phone and my computer. Do some research and come up with alternative activities and you will soon start to feel the benefits.

One great habit I have developed is to turn off my phone at least one hour before I go to bed. This habit has massively improved the quality of my sleep. Phones and other electric devices emit so-called blue light. Exposure to blue light from the sun during daytime hours is beneficial, it helps maintain a healthy circadian rhythm — your body's natural wake and sleep cycle — boosts alertness, helps memory and cognitive functions, and elevates your mood. So blue light itself is good for you, but blue light also messes with your body's ability to prepare for sleep. Blue light is responsible for blocking a hormone called melatonin. Melatonin is a natural hormone that makes you sleepy. By being exposed to blue light before going to bed you're less drowsy than usual at night and it takes you longer to fall asleep. Exposure to blue light before going to bed can have a detrimental influence on the quality of your sleep, resulting in a feeling of tiredness in the morning, which makes you feel like you haven't gotten enough sleep.

As you wake up in the morning, do not turn your phone on right away. Looking through your phone first thing in the morning is the worst way of starting your day. By doing that your mind starts the day by focusing on your phone and social media rather than on yourself and boosting your productivity. Your focus determines your reality, thus you should be asking yourself what you want to be focusing on. Avoid turning on your phone for the first 30 minutes that you are awake, in this way you will be able to shift the focus of the day towards yourself and your goals. It is very helpful for your mind and your awareness and allows you to practice self-discipline as well.

When you start your day you want to know exactly what you need to do and what you need to be working on, which is why you want to make sure to have a schedule and stick to it. Our body needs structure and routine in our lives. Our body performs best when we operate on a regular schedule. Most importantly, we need to eat and sleep about the same time each day not to mess up our circadian rhythm. This routine stays with a person their whole life and helps them develop good work habits. Find a schedule that works for you and stick to it. Effective time management is directly correlated with better academic or professional performances and lower anxiety levels. This is why large companies' CEOs usually have very interesting and unique routines and habits that allow them to squeeze the most out of their days. Bill Gates for instance, after he wakes up he takes 10 minutes to plan his whole day as accurately as possible, meaning he breaks down his day in five to ten minute-blocks and assigns every single block to a specific task. Our time in this world is limited, we do not have more than a certain amount. None of us know how much time we've left, and we cannot win any time back. Thus, you need to manage your own time as best as you can. You'll get what you focus on, so focus on what you want. Time is the most valuable asset you have, you want to make sure to make the best possible investment with it. How you leverage this resource will dictate your potential for success. Mastering effective time management needs to be on top of your to-do list.

When you try to schedule your day and figure out what you need to get done, it's important to focus on what's urgent and forget about the unnecessary things. Steve Jobs, Apple's co-founder, had an incredibly profound, yet simple morning routine. Each day he would get up, go through his routine, and then look himself in the mirror. He'd lock eyes with himself and ask, "If today was the last day of my life, would I be happy with what I'm about to do today?" If the answer was "No" for multiple days in a row, he knew he had to change something. Find the system that works best for managing your time and implement it. Once this habit has been solidified into your daily routine, virtually anything is possible, and no goal will be too big to attain.

Finding the most efficient way to complete your tasks allows you to value your precious time. Perfectionism is the worst disease for your time management.

Perfectionism ruins your time management and causes you to lose incredible amounts of time on irrelevant things. Perfectionism is the mother of procrastination. Instead of aiming for perfection, you should aim for "better than yesterday". I was a perfectionist myself; I would spend an enormous amount of time on every little task just to make it look perfect. I would worry about the tiniest most insignificant detail, trying to create a masterpiece. Eventually, this turned out to only be an enormous waste of time, since perfection is unreachable. There is no such thing as perfection in life. If you aim for perfection you have already failed before even starting. Vilfredo Pareto, an Italian engineer, sociologist, economist, political scientist, and philosopher came up with the so-called "80/20 Rule". Pareto's principle states that 80% of the results usually come from 20% of the work. Or, in other words, you want to focus on the 80% of your work, getting the most important part of it done, without caring about every little detail. That last 20% is what is going to cost you ridiculous amounts of time to complete and you won't gain any extra value from it. Thus, trying to make your project perfect, trying to reach 100% is first of all impossible, and secondly, extremely time-consuming. The pursuit of excellence is gratifying and healthy. The pursuit of perfection is frustrating, neurotic, and an incredible waste of time. Maximize your productivity by investing most of your time and energy on those specific tasks that will create the biggest impact. Once you've finished those tasks, you can focus on other activities that are on your to-do list. Following this principle will greatly improve your time management and will create much more time for you to focus on something else.

Being time efficient allows you to be able to invest your time in more activities, like taking time for yourself every now and then. It should be a primary concern of yours to make time for yourself and find clarity. The most important relationship is the one you have with yourself. Taking time for yourself is important for your health, your body, and your mental integrity. Your body needs some time off, where you rest on your couch, do what you love, and focus on feeling good and relaxed. Love yourself enough to set boundaries. Your own time and energy are precious. It's your choice how you invest them. A great way to do it is to take a full day for yourself, during which you wake up when you want, take care of your personal hygiene, watch a movie, or do what makes you feel good. This is a good way for your mind to shut off for one day, rest, and recover. Taking a day off greatly helps prevent burn-out or excessive stress as well.

Arriving on time is important to one's success. People always notice when you are late. Your punctuality is an indicator of whether you mean what you say and can be trusted, or you don't value commitments. You do not want people to think you don't value your commitment towards them by showing up later than expected. It will be beneficial for you and your professional, as well as personal relationships to create the habit of being punctual. You will never be punctual if you plan to get where you need to get at the scheduled time. Procrastination will kick in, unexpected delays will occur, and you will most likely end up being late. Always plan with a margin of at least fifteen minutes. If you need to leave the house by 8:00 a.m., then be ready to leave at least by 7:45 a.m. If you have some extra time left, you can do some chores around the house in the meantime, but most likely you will end up making your appointment just in time. In life you always need to be ahead of time, you need to be ahead of the game. You want to plan for every possible event that can happen next. Think about any possible delay or unforeseen circumstance that can show up and could cost you valuable time. Only in this way you can overcome difficulties and meet your deadlines in life. Being ahead of the game is a great strategy, which not only will relieve your stress, but is also a professional skill, which various jobs and businesses require you to have.

In your life, both in your professional, and in your personal life, you will come across other people. You will have to interact, confront yourself, or debate with thousands of people in your life. The way you approach and interact with other people can make a huge difference in your life and can allow you to build up hundreds of amazing relationships. The best guideline to follow when interacting with other people is the so-called "Golden Rule", "Do unto others as you would have them do unto you". It is a simple, yet effective principle to have in your life. Make this rule one of your principles and your relationships and conflict resolution abilities will improve so much. Respecting people of all races and beliefs is a hallmark of living life to the fullest. Acts of random kindness towards people that matter in your life help make the other person happier and make you feel great as well. You thereby show the other person that you value their presence in your life, while at the same time makes you feel good. Not only receiving can make one feel good, giving makes one feel exactly as good, if not better.

Money can't buy happiness. Money can't buy a happy family, true love, passion, time, respect, or inner peace. Consider yourself rich when counting all the things in your life that money cannot buy. Only then, when you understand that money is not all that matters, and that there are far more important things than money, will you truly be successful and happy in your life. Being successful in your life oftentimes means achieving your purpose, but how can you reach success and fulfillment if you are never grateful for what you have in the first place? It is so easy to get into the bad habit of envying what others have. Practice thinking about what you should be thankful for. The only strategy you have to stop focusing on your problems is to focus on what you have. Gratitude is a time-tested pathway to success, health, and happiness. It shifts your focus from what you lack to what you have, so from a negative standpoint to a positive one. Every successful person will tell you that you need to work on your mindset first and foremost in order to reach your goals and be successful.

Everybody has a different level of success, and everybody has a different level of contentment. When are you content with what you have? Is there a level of success you would be content with, or are you always striving for more? Most entrepreneurs are always striving for more. They get busier, they work harder and get more stressed. Take time to celebrate instead, take time off, and be content with what you have. That is true success right there. Acknowledging the good that you already have in your life is the foundation for all abundance. Only then you can pursue your goals in life. Write a daily list of things you're grateful for or make it a habit to say one thing you're grateful for when you sit down for dinner with your family. You will be so much happier with your life once you've learned to appreciate it and be grateful for it. Be grateful for every second of every day that you get to spend with the people you love. Life is short, and it's fragile. We don't know how many birthdays we have left. We don't need to have a birthday to celebrate, just celebrate life. If you haven't told someone you love them, do it. Do it now, tell people you love them. Call your friends, text them, hug them kiss them.

Your friend-group can have a massive influence on the way your life is going to develop. "Teamwork makes the dream work" is a common cliché, but you can turn it into a way of living. Yes, because surrounding yourself with the right people, will make a difference in your life. You do not want to be surrounded by partiers, stoners, and people who just want to have fun, otherwise, you are likely to end up like them. Surround yourself with people that are better than you, people which you can learn something from. People that make you work hard to keep up with them. Think about the people you have surrounded yourself with, then think about your goals and where you want to be in 10 years. Now look back at the people around you and ask yourself if they can help you getting where you want to get. If the answer is no, you probably want to reconsider your friends' group.

◆◆◆

"A small leak will sink a great ship", these are Benjamin Franklin's words. Your assets represent your ship, and your ship will be sunk if you don't learn to beware of your expenses. It's easy to lose sight of little expenses, but they can add up, especially if we don't budget. Budget and track your expenses to make sure you aren't wasting money you might need one day. See budgeting doesn't seem important until it's too late. Most people don't start to budget because they don't see the purpose of it, and they are right. There is no purpose for it as long as you are happy with your life the way it is, and are not seeking any improvement. The moment you realize the importance of budgeting is when you set a goal, a dream that you want to realize that is going to require some money. Let's say you have always wanted to start your own business and quit your current job. You would love to be able to become your own boss and enjoy the freedom associated with that. Well, starting your own business is going to require you a considerable investment, depending on the kind of business, it is going to take up a certain amount of your paycheck. At that point, you will have to start cutting corners everywhere, and it's not going to be easy. When you realize how hard it is to save up a lot of money in a short period of time, you will regret not having started saving earlier. On top of that, saving and beware of your expenses teaches you how to manage your personal finances in a better way. This will allow you to have more money on the side to spend or invest in your long-term goals, rather than waste it on short-term satisfaction.

To start budgeting you first of all need to work out your income. Put down all sources of income you have and their exact amount. Continue by working out your essential fixed price expenditures, which are fees, or bills that are unavoidable. To this, you add the essential variable price expenditures, which are food, clothes, and personal care. Now that you worked out these figures, you subtract these expenditures from your income, and the result hopefully turns out positive. If it doesn't however, cutting expenses any further is not an option anymore, thus you need to focus on increasing your income. There are multiple options for you to increase your income, depending on your personal situation you can find a second job, or invest in training and get a higher paying job. There are many more options available too, like freelancing, or self-employing. Assuming your income is higher than your essential expenditures the next step is to set up a contingency fund. A contingency fund is a set amount of money you put aside for unforeseen expenses, or for certain long-term investments you are planning to make. Unforeseen expenses will come up almost daily, thus a contingency fund is a must. There is no magical number you need to save, the recommendation is to save as much as possible of your income, at least 20%. This money should go into an instant access savings account, to have it readily available at all times. Finally, what's left of your income, only after having paid for all essentials and having rooted some money in your contingency fund, can be spent on luxuries, hobbies, entertainment, or other personal wishes.

Someone that can't keep track of their expenses cannot become successful, in the same way, that a leaking ship cannot sail across the ocean. Do not waste away your future, it's the only one you have.

THE BENEFITS
OF HAVING
GOOD HABITS

The Law of Hypnotic Rhythm is when a thought or physical movement is repeated over and over to the point where it reaches permanency. In other words, the more something is repeated, the more likely it is to get locked in motion. And when that happens it is incredibly difficult to change. The longer habits are in motion, the more power they have over you. That is why it is crucial to be aware of your habits and design them intentionally to change your lifestyle. The first step to take towards reaching any goal is to start and stick to a daily habit. If you want to run a marathon, you will have to start by running every day. If you want to be able to lift 200 pounds, you will have to lift weights every day for a long time. Good habits are the building blocks of success, master your habits and you can master your life. You will encounter a lot of obstacles, but ultimately that is what makes the journey fun: from nothing to something. Ultimately, you are what you say and what you do. Your habits will determine who you become and what habits you choose to follow will build the foundation for your life.

We are all writing a book. What does your book look like? Your life is a book, and you have a bunch of chapters in your book. But when they close that book, how good was that book? Was it worth writing it, or should you have written a different one?

Nothing comes from nothing. If you exercise every day, you become a healthy person. If you study every day you become an acculturated person. If you work hard, you will have a great return. Know what and who you want to be, and work towards that, by doing what you need to be doing. Once you are in your 70s you will look back at your life and will beat yourself up for all the time you wasted on irrelevant activities. Good habits reduce your time waste helping you to become a better person. There is always a better way of spending time than doing nothing. The sooner you learn to value your remaining time, the most you can make out of it.

Having good habits implemented in your life improves your mood remarkably. Good habits develop your mind and help you grow and be happier and healthier. Physical activity, for instance, stimulates the production of endorphins. Endorphins are brain chemicals that make you feel happier. Eating a healthy diet as well as exercising gets you in shape. You will feel better about your appearance, boosting your confidence and self-esteem. Think about all those days you lack motivation and you just can't get anything done. You just don't feel like exercising, going to work, or eating healthy. Developing habits makes it natural for your mind to have to exercise, eat healthily, etc. You don't have to force yourself anymore, it becomes the standard without constantly foraging for motivation.

Healthy habits are a valuable medicine for certain health conditions, such as heart diseases, strokes, and high blood pressure. Having a healthy lifestyle will spare you so many unpleasant surprises down the road. It can make the difference between feeling great all the way to your 90s and going through a painful and anticipated aging process. If you take care of yourself, you can keep your cholesterol and blood pressure within a safe range. This keeps your blood flowing smoothly, decreasing your risk of cardiovascular diseases. We've all experienced a lethargic feeling after eating too much junk food. When you eat a balanced diet, you give your body the fuel it needs to manage your energy levels optimally.

Regular physical exercise also improves muscle strength and boosts endurance, giving you more energy. Exercise also helps deliver oxygen and nutrients to your tissues and gets your cardiovascular system working more efficiently so that you have more energy to go through your daily activities. It also boosts your energy by promoting better sleep. This helps you fall asleep faster and get deeper sleep. Healthy habits generally boost your energy, allowing you to get through your days much easier, getting more work done, and most importantly helping you feel better and younger. When you practice healthy habits, you boost your chances to live a longer life. A study conducted by The American Council on Exercise showed that people who walked 30 minutes every day significantly reduced their chances of dying prematurely, compared with those who didn't exercise. The only habit of walking every day can allow you to have more time on this planet to spend with loved ones and do what you like, think about that!

Bad habits are hard to break, but once you adopt a healthier lifestyle, you won't regret this decision. You will feel much better and be much more comfortable with your own body.

The benefits are not only physical. It's on the mental level that good habits really make the difference. Success doesn't come by accident, it's a choice. It's a choice you make every day on and on, keeping up with your routines and working on your personal growth. The foundation for success is the mindset, no success is attainable unless you have the correct mindset. It's all in your head, and what's in your head will determine your success. Good habits further your personal growth and improve your mindset as you go.

"Whether you think you can, or you can't; You're right!"

Henry Ford

Train your mind to always think you can.

SUCCESSFUL PEOPLE'S HABITS

Good habits are the key to success. Your habits determine who you are and who you will become. Your habits help you develop your mind and your mindset, allowing you to improve yourself. Many successful people have their own routines and stick to certain good habits to be able to achieve extraordinary goals.

- Barack Obama -

Former US President Barack Obama, the first African-American US President spends his early hours preparing for his day. He prioritizes his beloved daughters, starting his day by having breakfast with them and his lovely wife Michelle, no matter how busy his day is. Barack Obama gets up at least two hours before his first scheduled meeting, which oftentimes means he needs to get up before 6:00 a.m. As soon as he gets out of bed, he hits the gym, doing cardio and aerobic exercises. After that, he reads the newspaper until 8:30 a.m. He then has a healthy breakfast with his whole family, before getting ready for work. Former President Obama is a hard worker, he usually works until quite late, most of the time past 11:30

p.m. After which he gets ready for bed, but before going to bed he likes to read something for half an hour. We can see from this routine how Barack Obama prioritizes the emotional and personal aspects of his routine, starting off the day among the people he loves, a great way of boosting his emotional energy before a hard day's work. He might have been the US President, but he's a father and husband first and foremost. He takes his personal time and his duty as a father and husband seriously. He spends a lot of time exercising and meditating to improve his productivity and his mindset.

- Elon Musk -

Elon Musk, Tesla's and Space X's owner, has a quite different vision of the day. He usually gets up at 7:00 a.m. after only six hours of sleep. He spends the first half an hour of his day addressing critical emails. Musk likes to drink coffee in the morning, which wakes him up and gives him more awareness. Surprisingly, he does not eat breakfast, even though eating a healthy breakfast is known to be very beneficial. A day is a lemon to be squeezed for Musk. A waterfall of commitments and meetings that await him. For him, it's all about prioritizing what's important. His average week is made up of 85 to a staggering 100 hours of work. Musk has a quite interesting way to schedule his week: from Tuesday to Thursday he commits himself to Tesla, and on Mondays and Fridays, he works on Space X. Tesla, his successful electric car company, takes up most of his working hours, usually adding up to at least 42 hours a week. Space X, on the other hand, is his space travel company. Musk tries to cut edges everywhere to make up some extra time. He doesn't waste any time answering calls and uses a secret email to avoid being contacted. Fun fact, he usually eats in the middle of meetings, in no more than five minutes. At least he gives himself enough time for dinner, during which, he admitted, he eats a lot.

Elon Musk's routine is quite unique and stressful. Undoubtedly, his goal is to squeeze the maximum hours out of his days. He fully dedicates himself to his job, which is the best part of this routine. He doesn't waste any time on things he doesn't deem relevant to his goals. On the other hand, this routine is incredibly demanding for his body and might not be the best way to go for his health and well-being, but certainly does make him very productive and effective.

- Bill Gates -

Another well-known American billionaire is William Henry Gates III, better known as Bill Gates, owner, and co-founder of Microsoft Corporation. Bill Gates kickstarts his day with some good exercise. Gates is known for spending the first hour of his mornings running on the treadmill, which improves his cognition and focus throughout the day. Waking up early to exercise also enhances his self-discipline, which is likely to affect other areas of Gates' life. Gates likes to break down his day to the minute. No matter how wealthy he is, his most valuable possession will always be his remaining time alive, he said.

This is why he doesn't want to waste any minute of his life and schedules every day meticulously. He tries to be as efficient as possible, avoiding wasting too much time on any activity, thereby keeping his productivity high. Bill Gates is a life-long learner. Despite being 65 years of age and being a multi-billionaire, he dedicates at least one hour a day to improve his knowledge, learning about any deliberate topics. He's known to read about 50 books a year. Benjamin Franklin once said, "An investment in knowledge pays the best interest.", which clearly applies to Bill Gates and everyone out there committed to improving themselves. Quite interestingly Gates still does his own dishes. Daily tasks like these are a great way to practice mindfulness and promote calmness and creativity. This proves how it's all about mindset. If you get in the right mindset, even chores can be valuable opportunities. Gates invests a lot of time in himself and his well-being. He values his sleep particularly and makes sure that he goes to bed early enough to snag at least seven hours of sleep. Lack of sleep not only impairs your cognitive processes, such as attention, alertness, and problem-solving, but it also leads to heart diseases and high blood pressure.

Gates' approach and vision of life, seems the total opposite of Elon Musk's, yet proves to be extremely successful. Although you may not be striving to become one of the richest people on earth or building a giant software company, you can definitely see the benefits of building your own routines.

- Mark Zuckerberg -

Mark Zuckerberg, a successful internet entrepreneur, and Facebook's co-founder and CEO, has yet another way of boosting his productivity. With his minimalist approach of wearing the same clothes every day, he avoids wasting his first thoughts in the morning on what to wear and focuses instead on his business. "I try to make as few decisions as possible about anything except how to best serve this community.", says Zuckerberg. He wears sports jeans, sneakers, and a gray t-shirt every day.

- Arnold Schwarzenegger -

Few people in the world are so dedicated to success and work as hard to achieve their goals as Arnold Schwarzenegger does. The Austrian-American actor, retired professional bodybuilder, and former Governor of California is a true example for many people. His mindset has allowed him to build up an impeccable career and worldwide fame. One of the many secrets to his success was meditation. Meditation has helped him a great deal to fight against anxiety over the years. He would often get lost in his worries and would struggle to overcome such thoughts until he started meditating. Moreover, daily meditation is a great tool not to lose sight of your path towards success, it can help you find your purpose and stay motivated. To combat pressure, Schwarzenegger breaks down his schedule into sessions: 45 to 60 minutes of diligent work and concentration, followed by a break. During this time, quite interestingly, he likes to play chess or work out, in order to stimulate different parts of his brain. Most people are more productive in short stints, rather than over long hauls, making this a great philosophy. In his book, Schwarzenegger talked about competition and how his perspective on competition completely changed after a crushing defeat by bodybuilder Chet Yorton. Instead of constantly comparing himself to others or basing his success on beating someone else, he decided to shift his focus towards his personal goals, without trying to be better, or stronger than anyone. Psychologists support this mindset, as those who always compare themselves to others don't understand the value of improving and developing their own talents and skills. The only person you should strive to be better than, is the person you were yesterday.

If you now look at all these successful people, or even at other world-leading entrepreneurs, they all have very different routines and habits, yet they all tend to get up early, stay focused, and work very hard. The point is you don't need the exact same routine as Bill Gates or Elon Musk, but you need A routine and stick with it. What routine you want to make yours is up to you but get used to follow certain good habits and take control of your life.

THE 30-DAY CHALLENGE

You have to have goals outside of your comfort zone that will challenge you because, in order to do something you've never done, you have to become someone you've never been.

A 30-Day Challenge is a proven strategy to effectively implement new healthy habits in your life. It's a way to try new habits and take up new challenges without putting the pressure of a long-time commitment on yourself. Habit building requires consistency, which is oftentimes hard to maintain. Having a fixed time span will greatly boost your motivation and work ethic, as you can clearly visualize your time-goal. Persisting for 30 days at your challenge seems far easier than "persisting for life". The desire to change yourself permanently is filled with a lot of pressure and self-doubt. A wise person once said, "Self-doubt kills more dreams than failure ever will". You cannot expect to be able to change yourself and your lifestyle overnight, this is a long-term process, which requires discipline and dedication. There are all kinds of challenges you can experiment with, for successfully getting your life under control, taking better care of your health, or to overcome procrastination. Trying a 30-Day Challenge is an absolute must. You will notice the influence it has on your life already after the first try, and the fulfillment you experience when you complete your first 30-Day Challenge is indescribable. Completing such challenges will have a massive influence on your self-esteem and your self-discipline. It's a way to get control over your body and its actions. Moreover, after completing your 30-Day Challenge, chances are you might even stick to the new behavioral pattern, successfully implementing it in your daily life. On top of that, setting a fixed time span is a great way to find out what works for you and what doesn't. It's a short enough time to be able to experiment with many different challenges, yet long enough to see how it affects your life, both physically and emotionally. At the end of a 30-Day Challenge, you most often have a clear idea of how your new habit influenced your life. If things are going in the direction you expected them to go, you can keep up with your new habit, if not, you can always try something else, until you find the right fit for you.

A great idea for a 30-Day Challenge is not to eat anything sweet or not to drink anything but water. Other valuable options are to keep a daily journal, meditate, or read every day. If you want to work on your body instead, 100 push-ups a day is the perfect challenge for you. Experiment with intermittent fasting, no mobile phone, or no TV to learn not to give in to temptations. If you want to work on your mindset and focus, I would suggest not to watch any news. Lastly, if you want to improve your work ethic you should try to learn a new language in 30 days. These are only a few ideas for your first 30 Day Challenge, but you can find many more on the web.

Now the time for you to act has come. Choose your 30-Day Challenge and start now. Take full control of your life and discover the immense potential of your body and mind. The journey will be tough, do not get frustrated by obstacles and problems along the way, but try to look at them as a chance to grow and improve yourself. You know the concept, you have multiple options for your first 30 Day Challenge, so the only thing left is to start your challenge. I ask you, for your own sake and the good of your future, to stop procrastinating and start acting. Get a calendar, pick the challenge you want, and cross the first day out of the calendar. All the opportunities you need in your life are right here in front of you, you only need to get up from your couch and take them.

◆◆◆

Wrapping up, there is so much to benefit from good habits in your life. The right habits can add value to your life and help you become the person you've always wanted. It all comes down to you and your willpower. You need to decide what you want to do with your life, you need to find the motivation to start acting yourself. With the right motivation, mindset, and dedication you can and will be able to master all your habits. And when you fail, do not be disappointed. Failing is part of the process. What were you expecting? To succeed without not even failing once? Even the people that have been doing this for years keep making mistakes on a regular basis. There is no losing, only learning; there is no failure, only opportunities; there are no problems, only solutions. Failure is the mother of all successes. Learn not to judge yourself or feel guilty for your mistakes but use your mistakes as a lesson and get back on track again. And if on a rare and unfortunate occasion you skip one day of your new routine, make absolutely sure never to miss twice in a row. Let's be clear, you shouldn't miss any day, but if you happen to miss anyways, missing the second day in a raw means to restart from the beginning, throwing away all your efforts. Slipping up on your habits doesn't make you a failure, it makes you normal. What separates successful people from the others is they get back on track quickly.

Once you've fully developed your new healthy habit it will last a lifetime! The quicker you'll develop healthy habits, the better your life will become. Our life is the most precious thing we've got, why waste it away? As soon as you learn to invest in yourself and take care of your body and mind, you are set for success. Now it's up to you, make your time count, make your life a remarkable one.

CONCLUSION

Dear reader, congratulations for having read the entire book, I sincerely hope you enjoyed it and learned many great lessons from it. I once again want to express my gratitude to you for purchasing "Habits For Success" and hope it helped you find the motivation to take control of your life. The next step for you now is to use the acquired information to improve your quality of life and build the future you've always wanted.

If you enjoyed this book and feel like it added some extra value to your life, I kindly ask you to leave a quick review on Amazon. Your review would help me enormously to promote this emerging book and allow other people to benefit from its value. So please, feel free to leave a review on Amazon and share this book with your friends and family. If you are disappointed with this book feel free to share your thoughts as well, I would be happy to learn from your critique and improve myself and my book.

If you found value in this book, and want to keep improving yourself I encourage you to follow us on social media. We share great content on our platforms, from daily motivational quotes, blog articles about personal growth, to mindblowing speeches that will help you improve your mindset, guide you through your journey of personal growth and help you become a successful person.

YOU CAN FIND US HERE:

Facebook: @MissionLifeQuality

Instagram: @missionlifequality

Twitter: @MissionLifeQua1

TikTok: @missionlifequality

YouTube: @Mission Life Quality

If you want to reach out to us, you can contact us at the following e-mail address:

missionlifequality@gmail.com

To your freedom and success,

Mission Life Quality

"We are our own potters; for our habits make us, and we make our habits."

Frederick Langbridge

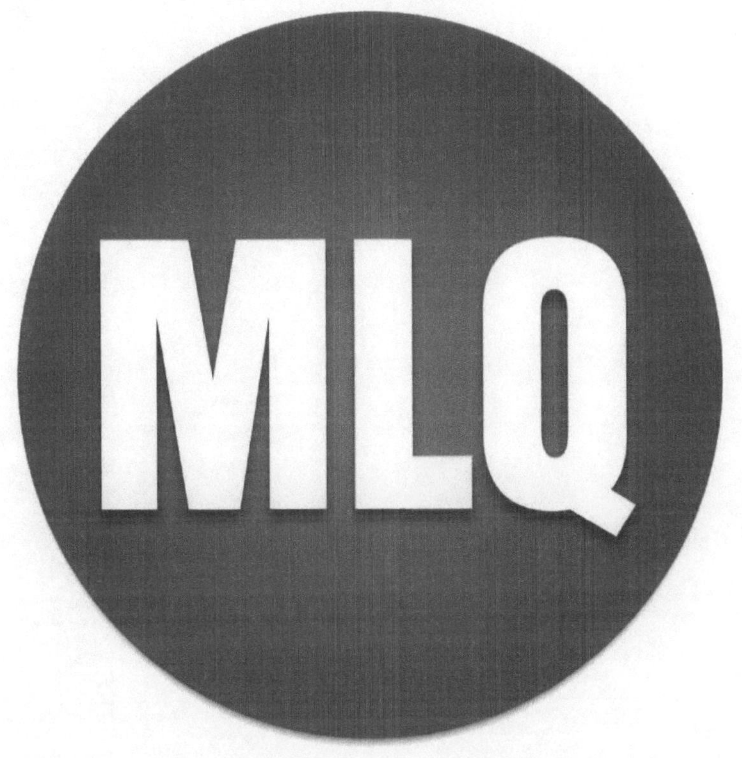

MISSION LIFE QUALITY

A brand devoted to the best quality of life, through a healthy nutrition, personal growth and much more.